Bartosz Chmielnicki

Pulse Qualities in Chinese Medicine at a Glance

Bartosz Chmielnicki

Pulse Qualities in Chinese Medicine at a Glance

With 32 illustrations

KIENER

Title of the original edition
Jakości Pulsu, Compleo, Katowice, Polen, first published in 2012;
1. English edition: Pulse Qualities, Compleo, Katowice, Poland

Notice
Neither the publisher nor the author assumes any responsibility for any loss or injury and/or damage to persons arising out of or related to any use of the material contained in this book. It is the responsibility of the treating practitioner, relying on independent expertise and knowledge of the patient, to determine the best treatment and method of application for the patient.

Bibliographic Information
A catalog record of this book is available from the British Library (www.bl.uk) and the Deutsche Nationalbibliothek (www.dnb.de).

Translation from German into English: Pia Huber, London
Copy-editing: Lisa Lorz, Bayreuth
Layout designer: Kadja Gericke, Herrenberg
Printer: Drukarnia Dimograf, Bielsko-Biała/Poland
Illustrations: Marta Szudyga; Zofia Oslislo, Katowice (Icons);
Henriette Rintelen, Velbert (p. 9)
Cover design: SpieszDesign, Neu-Ulm

ISBN 978-3-943324-84-6

www.kiener-press.com

Table of contents

Preface

A few years ago, I decided to teach pulse diagnosis at the Compleo school of TCM in Katowice, Poland. While I was preparing for the course, I realized that there would be two major problems trying to convey this information. One of them is related to nomenclature and the student's unfamiliarity with the Chinese characters of the acupuncture point names and the second is the difficulty to memorize 28 pulse descriptions. Realizing this created a desire in me to teach pulse characterisation in a way that would lead to a thorough understanding of the basic pulse qualities in each and every student.

After some reflection, I realized that I could portray the Chinese characters as symbolic cartoon-like pictures that resemble the basic characteristics of each pulse. A snake, which is similar in shape to a blood vessel, became the character of the pulses.

This is neither a manual nor a book about pulses. It is simply a quick tool that is helpful while learning basic pulse qualities. Those who seek more profound knowledge about Chinese pulse diagnosis should read the following texts:

- Sean Walsh, Emma King: "Pulse Diagnosis: A Clinical Guide"

- Qiao Yi, Al Stone: "Traditional Chinese Medicine Diagnosis Study Guide"

- Yang Shou-Zhong: "The Pulse Classic: A Translation of the Mai Jing"

I would like to especially recommend Frances Turners electronic publication "Chinese Pulse Images". Most of the Chinese name descriptions used in the following booklet are based on her explanations.

Bartosz Chmielnicki

Pulse on the radial artery

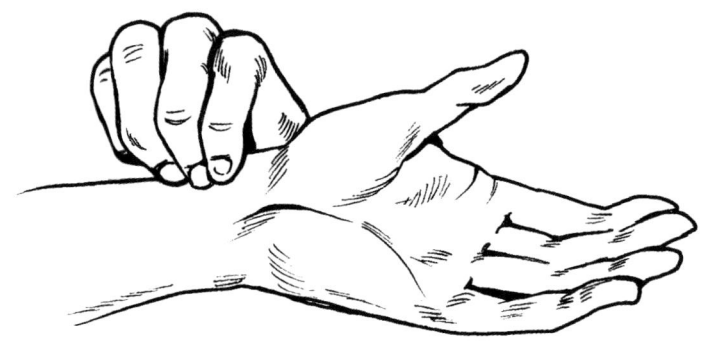

There are three positions for pulse examination:

→ *cun* – distal: reflects the state of the Upper Burner

→ *guan* – middle (at the level of the radial styloid process): reflects the state of the Middle Burner

→ *chi* – proximal: reflects the state of the Lower Burner

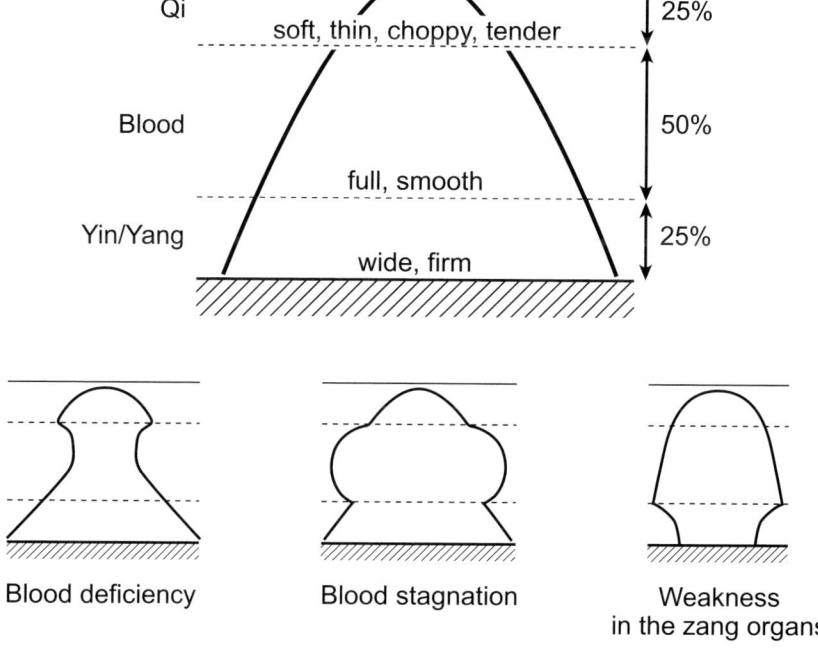

Blood deficiency   Blood stagnation   Weakness in the zang organs

… three levels of pulse examination:

→ superficial: reflects the state of Qi

→ middle: reflects the state of Blood

→ deep: reflects the state of internal organs

How to correctly examine the pulse

Place your middle finger at the level of the radial styloid process of your patient and index and ring fingers above and below it, respectively.

Feel the pulse with all three fingers on these positions with the aim to get a general impression of the pulse. The first level where you feel the pulse will be the superficial level.

Press the pulse to the level of full occlusion, when you feel bone under your fingertips. Then gently release the pressure; the first moment of feeling the pulse again will be the deep level.

Slowly releasing the pressure, lift your fingers back to the superficial level feeling the middle level between them.

Firstly name your general impression of the pulse – is it easily or hardly palpable, strong or weak, fast or slow, does volume or wall tension clearly dominate?

Then aim to precisely determine its:
→ width
→ depth
→ length
→ strength
→ wall tension
→ speed
→ rhythm
→ wave contour

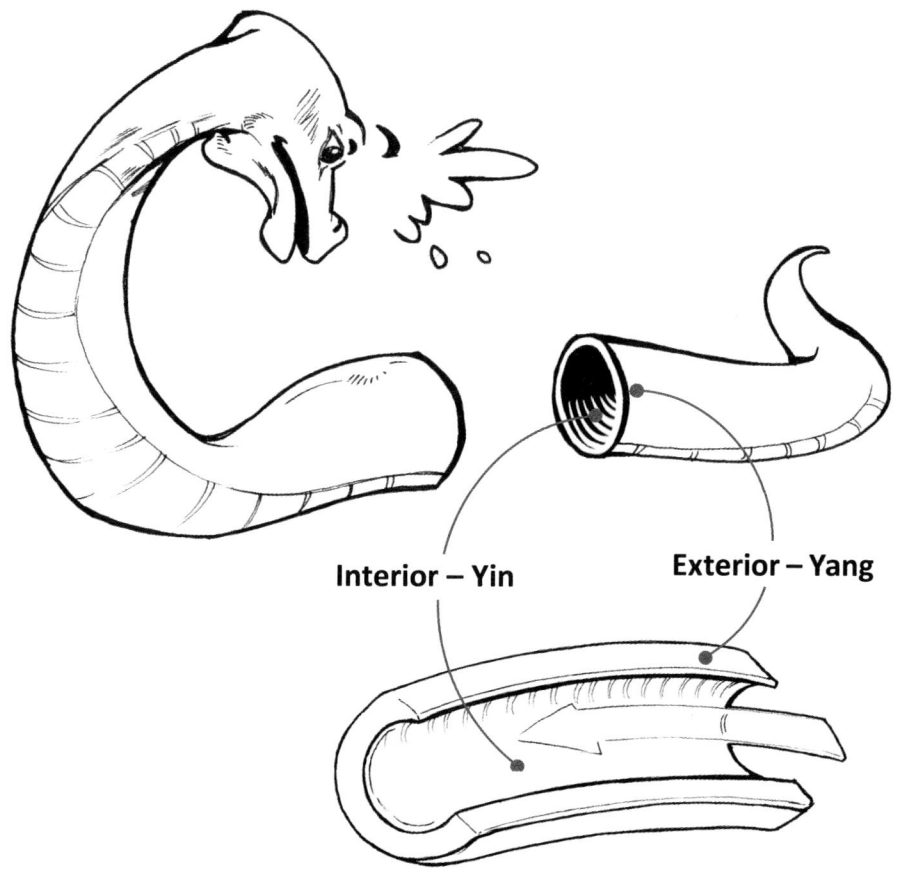

Interior – Yin   Exterior – Yang

Qi and Yang are manifested in the tension of the vessel wall, while the filling of the vessel reflects the state of Jinye, Blood and Yin.

Normal pulse

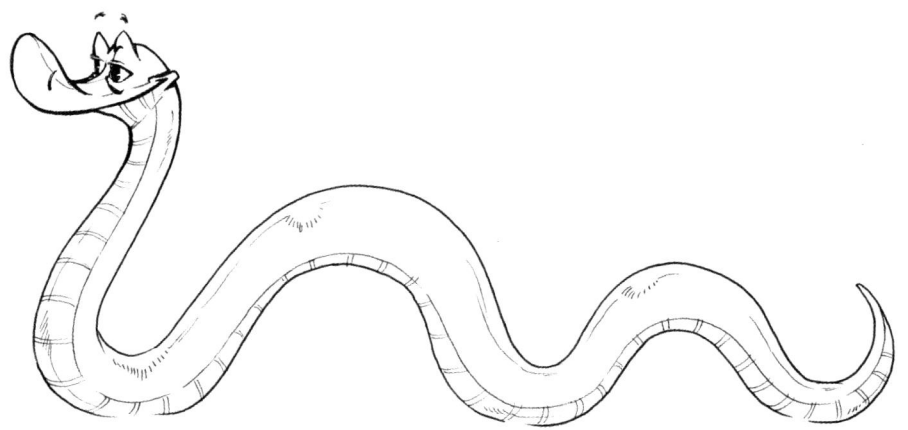

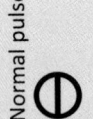

Width

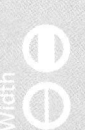

Length

Depth

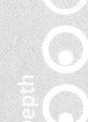

Speed

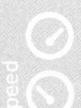

Rhythm

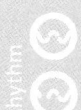

Strength

Vessel wall tension

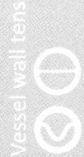

Three classic qualities of a normal pulse:

- It has good Stomach Qi: This describes the force of the pulse wave flowing under the fingertips and depends on interaction of Qi and Blood.

- It has good Shen: This means it is calm, regular and characterized by constant frequency, and appropriate force.

- It is rooted: There is a strong, rooted pulse felt on the *chi*-position, at the deep level (close to the bone).

Wave contour

slippery

choppy

overflowing

stirring

Width

The state of Qi, Blood and fluids is reflected by the width of the pulse.

◑ Increased width

Increased width has the following causes:

- The vessel is distended from inside by excessive heat ⎫
- Yin deficiency leads to Yang excess ⎬ Yang hyperactivity ⎭

- Presence of excesses of Yin

Pulses characterized by increased width:

➜ *shimai*

➜ *laomai*

➜ *hongmai*

➜ *jinmai* (slightly trembling)

➜ *gemai*

➜ *koumai*

➜ *sanmai*

➜ *huamai* (slightly slippery feeling)

➜ *xumai*

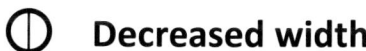 Decreased width

Decreased width is caused by deficiency of Yin aspects.

Pulses characterized by decreased width:

→ *ximai*

→ *weimai*

→ *rumai*

→ *ruomai*

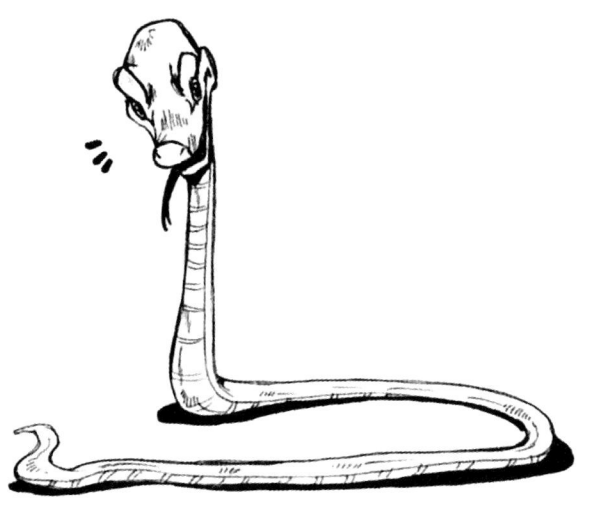

Normal pulse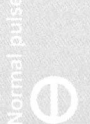

Width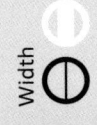

Length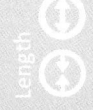

Depth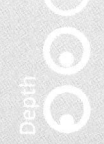

Speed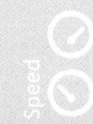

Rhythm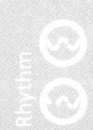

Strength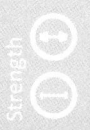

Vessel wall tension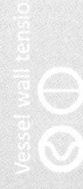

細脈　*xìmài* – Thin, silk-like pulse

Analysis of the character 細 *xì*

Consists of two parts.

- Left: 糸 *mi* or *si,* shows a thin thread
- Right: phonetic component
- Character as a whole: 'thin, silk-like'

Characteristics

The left part of the pulse name – thin thread – describes what can be palpated with the fingers.

Causes

A thin pulse may be formed in cases of deficiency of Yin, Blood and fluids, when the vessel cannot be filled up.

A thin pulse may also indicate constriction of the vessel by surrounding Dampness.

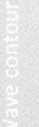

Wave contour

slippery

choppy

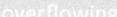

overflowing

stirring

Depth

Blood follows the movement of Qi. The localization of bodily processes and the state of the Yang aspect of Qi are reflected by the depth of the pulse.

◐ Superficial pulse

A superficial pulse indicates Qi and Blood moving towards the body surface:

- Attack of external pathogen – Wei Qi is fighting with a pathogen at the surface
- Yin deficiency – uncontrolled Yang moves to the surface

Superficial pulses, that can be palpated at the surface:

→ *fumai*

→ *shimai*

→ *gemai*

→ *koumai*

→ *sanmai*

→ *rumai*

⊙ Deep pulse

A deep pulse indicates that Qi and Blood cannot reach the body surface:
- Qi and Blood are blocked by a deeply penetrating, external pathogen
- Yang Qi and Blood deficiency

Deep Pulses:

→ *chenmai*

→ *fumai*

→ *laomai*

→ *ruomai*

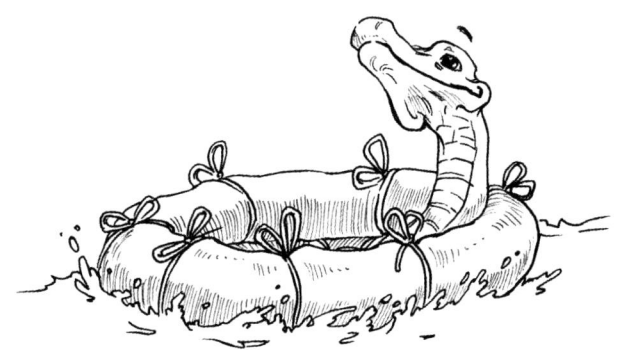

Normal pulse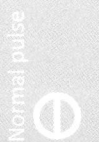

Width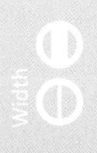

Length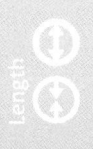

Depth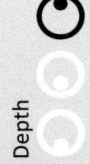

Speed

Rhythm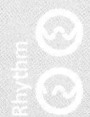

Strength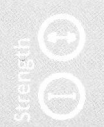

Vessel wall tension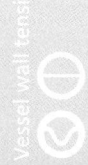

浮脈 *fúmài* – Floating pulse

Analysis of the character 浮 *fú*

Consists of two parts.

- Left: reduced form of 水 *shui* = water
- Right: 孚 *fu* = trust, confidence; hand of a mother protecting her child
- Character as a whole: image of a floating nest in which a bird looks after its brood

Characteristics

The Floating Pulse is strongest at the superficial level, and weakens with increased finger pressure, but is still palpable.

Causes

A Floating Pulse indicates the presence of pathogens blocking Yang Qi at the surface.

Yin deficiency makes Yang Qi unrooted, ascending to the surface, which is shown by a floating, accelerated, thin pulse.

Wave contour

slippery

choppy

overflowing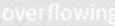

stirring

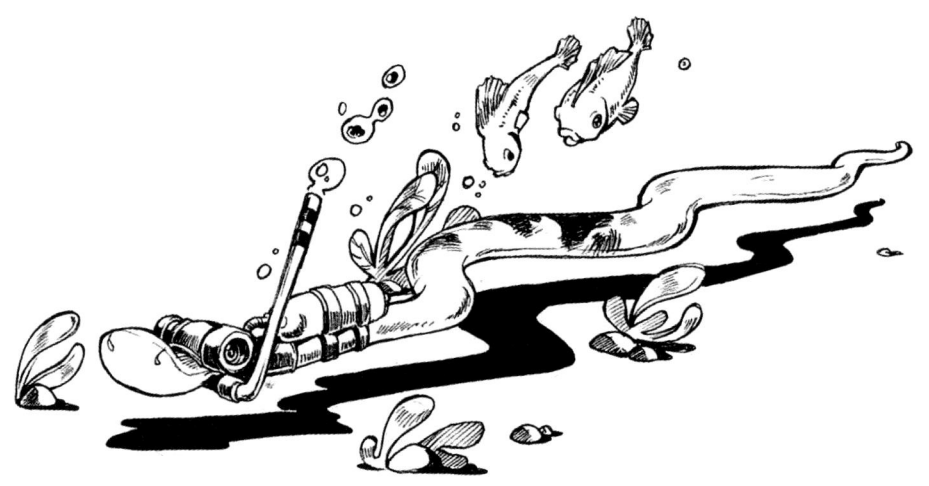

Normal pulse

Width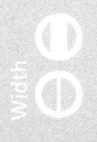

Length

Depth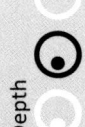

Speed

Rhythm

Strength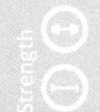

Vessel wall tension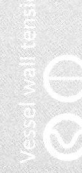

沉脉 *chénmài* – **Deep pulse**

Analysis of the character 沉 *chén*

Consists of two parts.

- Left: reduced form of 水 *shui* = water
- Right: 冗 *rong* = man or small table under a roof or under a covering
- Character as a whole: place covered by water with the meaning of 'deep'

Characteristics

A Deep pulse is felt strongest at the deep level.

Causes

The state of Yang Qi is reflected by the pulse depth; a deep pulse may occur when there is Yang Qi deficiency.

Yang Qi may also be bound inside by deep penetrating pathogens. In that case, a deep pulse points to stagnation.

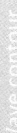

Wave contour

slippery

choppy

overflowing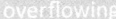

stirring

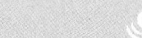

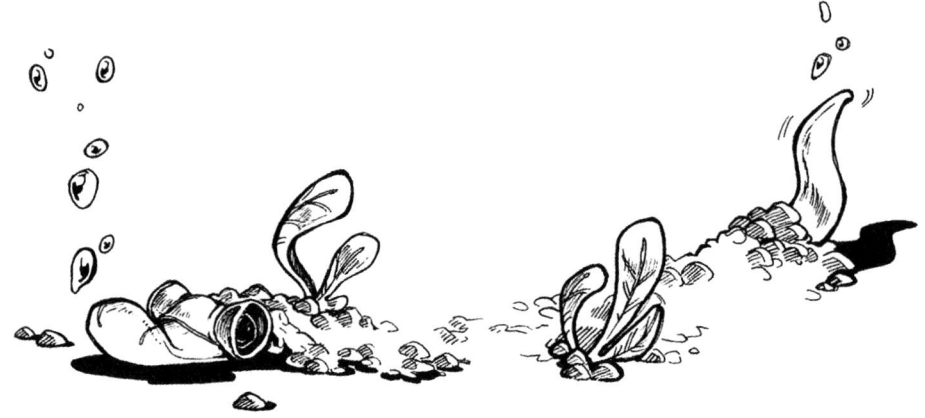

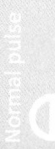

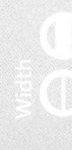

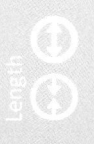

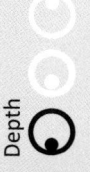

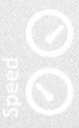

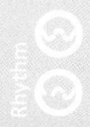

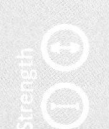

Normal pulse

Width

Length

Depth

Speed

Rhythm

Strength

Vessel wall tension

伏脈 *fúmài* – Hidden pulse

Analysis of the character 伏 *fú*

Consists of two parts.

- Left: reduced form of 人 *ren* = man

- Right: 犬 *quan* = dog

- Character as a whole: description of a situation in which a person imitates a dog, crawling like a soldier hiding from enemies

Characteristics

The hidden pulse is felt only at the deep level (just above the bone). It may be considered as a progression from the deep pulse.

Causes

This pulse is found in more serious illnesses than the deep pulse, but is mainly related to the state of the Yang energy:

- If it is hidden and weak, this indicates a severe Yang deficiency (and the associated cold).

- If it is hidden and strong, this indicates a severe stagnation of the Yang energy deep inside the body, which can be caused by an external pathogen or deep-seated stagnation (of food, Phlegm, toxic Heat, Heat due to internal hyperactivity of the Wei Qi).

Wave contour

slippery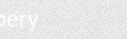

choppy

overflowing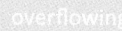

stirring

Length

The Length of the pulse is a function of Yang Qi.

⬍ Increased length

The increased length is caused by hyperactivity of the Yang-Qi.

Long pulse:

→ *changmai*

✪ Decreased length

A shorter length is due to the following factors:
- Qi deficiency
- Pathogen blocking the vessel

Short pulses:
→ *duanmai*

→ *dongmai*

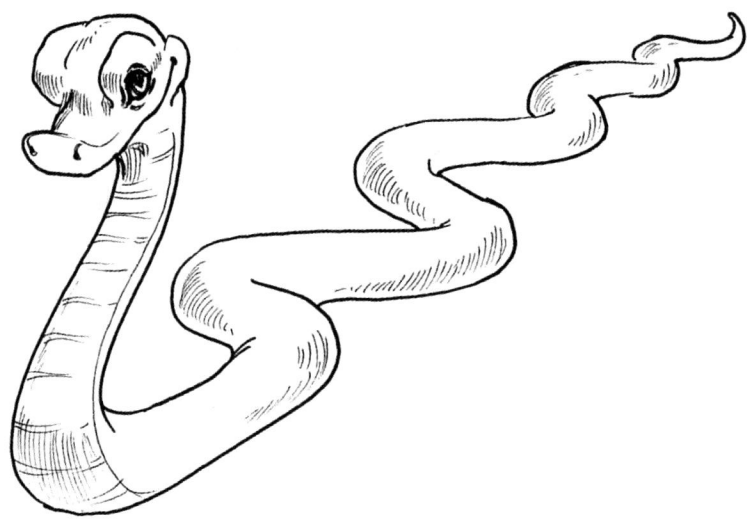

Normal pulse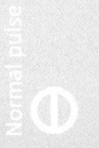

Width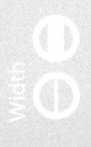

Length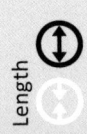

Depth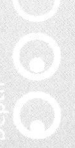

Speed

Rhythm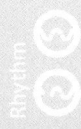

Strength

Vessel wall tension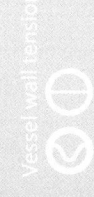

長脈 *chángmài* – Long pulse

Analysis of the character 長 *cháng*

Has its origin in an early pictogram that shows a man with long hair.

Characteristics

The long pulse is felt at all three positions, and behind the *chi* and/or *cun* position.

Causes

It may indicate a good state of health, or it may be present when there is excess of Yang, such as Heat or Liver Yang rising.

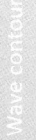

slippery

choppy

overflowing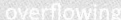

stirring

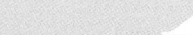

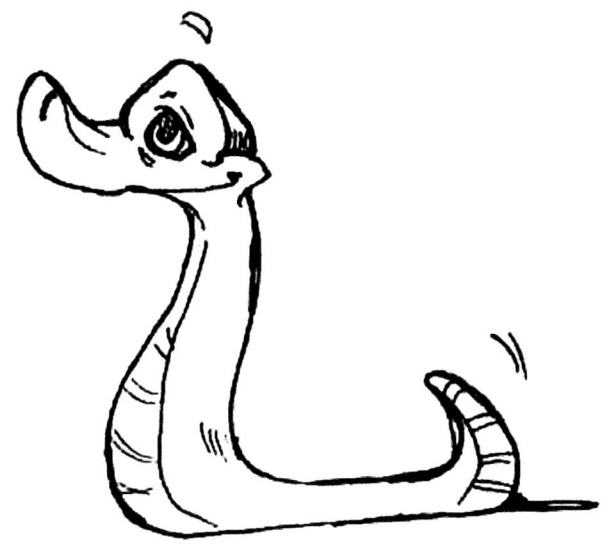

Normal pulse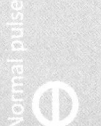

Width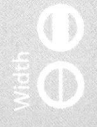

Length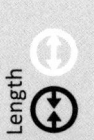

Depth

Speed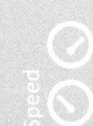

Rhythm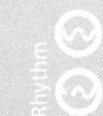

Strength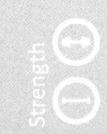

Vessel wall tension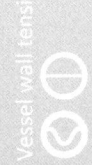

短脈 *duǎnmài* – Short pulse

Analysis of the character 短 *duǎn*

Consists of two parts.

- Left: 矢 *shi* = arrow (short shape of the spear)
- Right: 豆 *dou* = food in a jar or bean
- Character as a whole: a collection of short objects

Characteristics

Short pulses can be felt at least at one position.

Causes

A Short pulse is present when there is Qi stagnation resulting from Qi deficiency, or excesses.

Wave contour

slippery   choppy   overflowing   stirring

Strength

The strength of the pulse reflects vitality of Qi.

⊕ Increased strength

The increased strength is due to the following factors:
- Wei Qi fights with a pathogen
- Qi and Blood stagnation

Strong pulses:

→ *shimai*

→ *laomai*

→ *jinmai*

→ *dongmai*

→ *hongmai*

⊖ **Decreased strength**

Qi and Blood deficiency are reflected in decreased strength.

Weak pulses:

→ *xumai*

→ *weimai*

→ *rumai*

→ *ruomai*

→ *semai*

→ *sanmai*

→ *koumai*

→ *gemai*

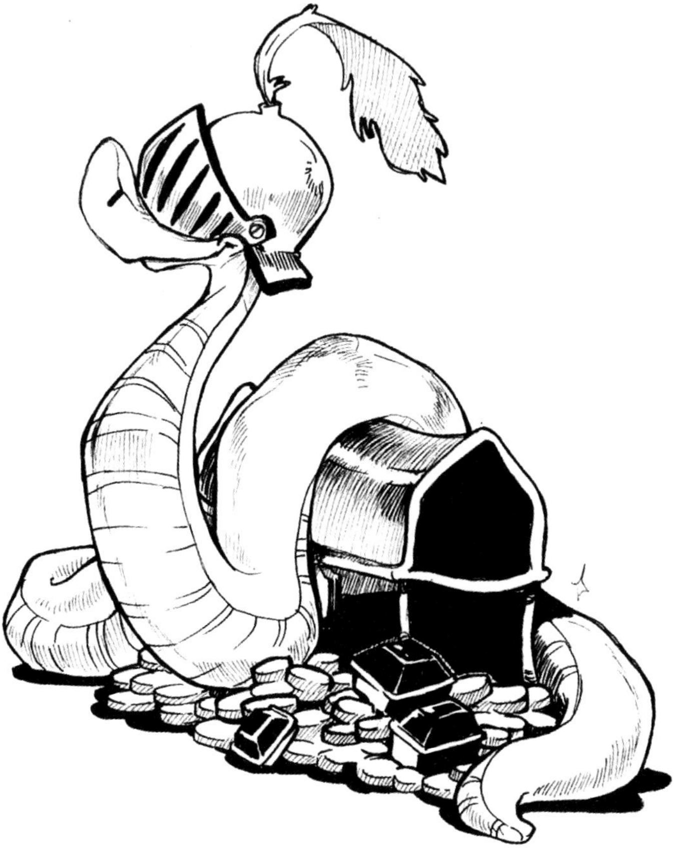

34

Normal pulse

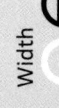
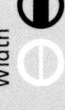
Width

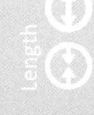
Length

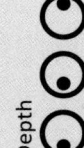
Depth

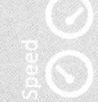
Speed

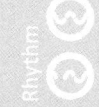
Rhythm

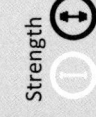
Strength

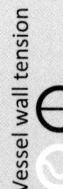
Vessel wall tension

實脈 *shímài* – Full pulse

Analysis of the character 實 *shí*

- Above: roof
- Below: a string with coins and cowrie shells
- Character as a whole: a treasury full of goods; substantial, stable, firm. In ancient China, cowrie shells were used as a currency.

Characteristics

- Increased strength
- Increased wall tension
- Increased width
- Being felt at all three levels

Causes

The full pulse results from a struggle between strong Wei Qi and a strong pathogen. It may also reflect the presence of intensified Heat syndrome (toxic, stagnated, etc.).

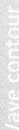

Wave contour

| slippery | choppy | overflowing | stirring |

  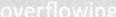

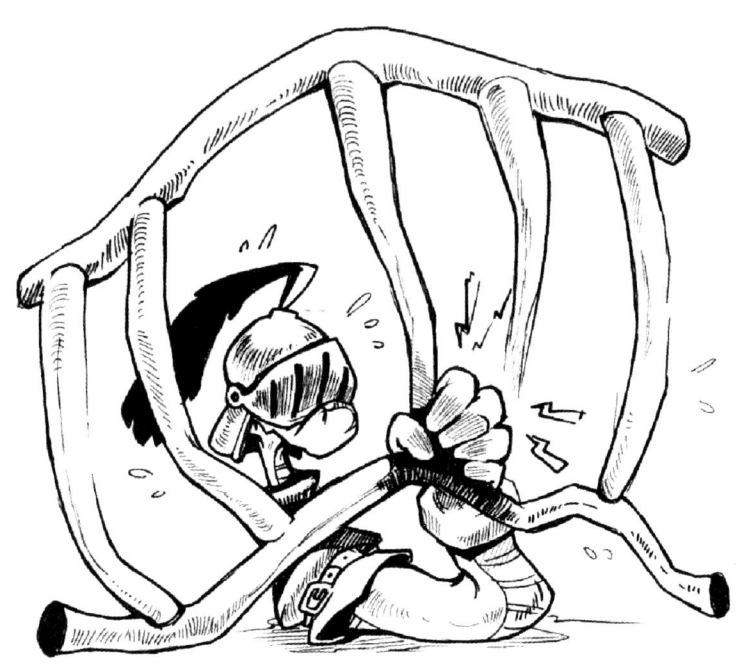

Normal pulse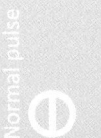

Width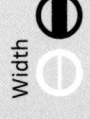

Length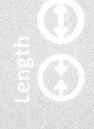

Depth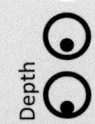

Speed

Rhythm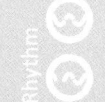

Strength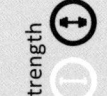

Vessel wall tension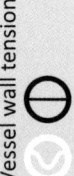

牢脈 *láomài* – Confined pulse

Analysis of the character 牢 *láo*

- Above: roof

- Below: ox or cow

- Character as a whole: ox or cow penned up in a cowshed. This picture is reminiscent of a great force that remains inside.

Characteristics

- Increased strength

- Increased wall tension

- Increased width

- Being felt at the deep level

Causes

A confined pulse results from the struggle between Wei Qi and a pathogen, which takes place deep inside. That situation may happen when an external pathogen penetrates inside, but may also be a result of direct invasion of Cold, for example into the Intestines or the Uterus.

Wave contour

slippery    choppy   overflowing 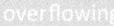   stirring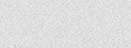

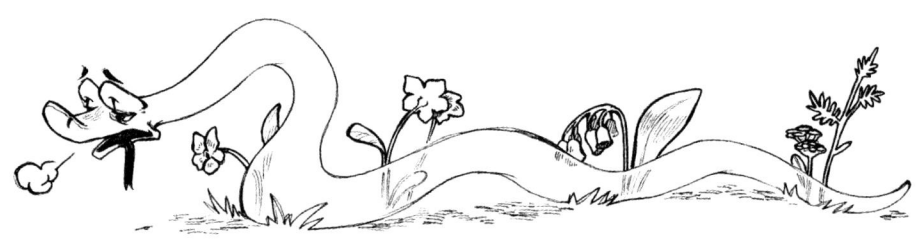

Normal pulse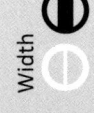

Width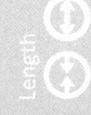

Length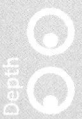

Depth

Speed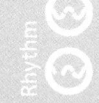

Rhythm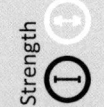

Strength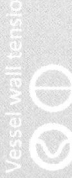

Vessel wall tension

虚脉 *xūmài* – **Empty pulse**

Analysis of the character 虚 *xū*

- Above: tiger

- Below: hill

- Character as a whole: shows a tiger lying on a hill. Tigers live in the wilderness. Wild, barren land contains nothing, which is why this character depicts emptiness.

Characteristics

The Empty pulse is easily occluded by increased finger pressure.

Causes

This pulse indicates Qi deficiency.

Wave contour

| slippery | choppy | overflowing | stirring |

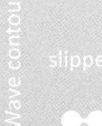

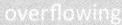

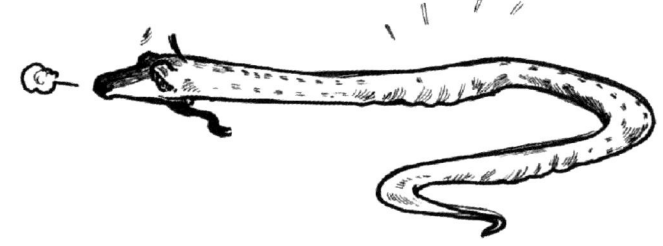

Normal pulse

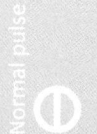

Width

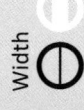

Length

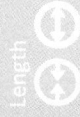

Depth

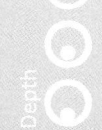

Speed

Rhythm

Strength

Vessel wall tension

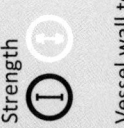
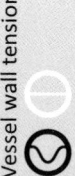

微脈 *wēimài* – Faint pulse

Analysis of the character 微 *wēi*

Consists of three parts.

- Left: the radical for 'walk'

- In the middle: a plant

- Right: a hand holding a stick

- Character as a whole: the plant is cut up into thin fibers that you can barely feel

Characteristics

The faint pulse can be barely felt:

- is very weak, almost undetectable

- is thin

- has a much decreased wall tension

- may be occluded even with very delicate pressure

Causes

A faint pulse indicates severe, long-lasting Qi and Blood deficiencies, but may also result from shock (Yang collapse).

slippery   choppy   overflowing   stirring

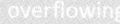

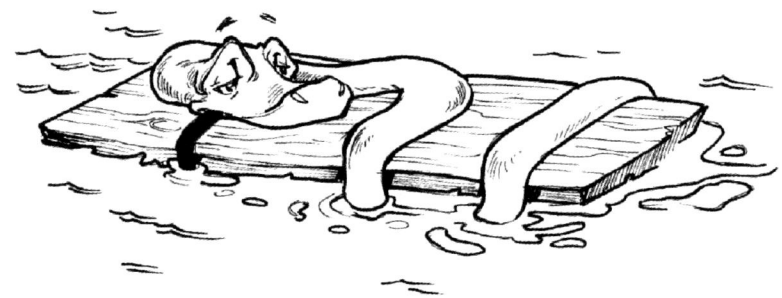

Normal pulse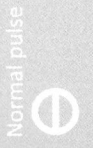

Width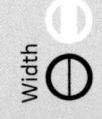

Length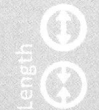

Depth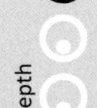

Speed

Rhythm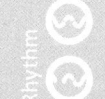

Strength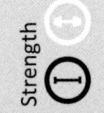

Vessel wall tension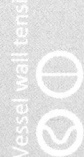

濡脈 *rúmài* – Soggy pulse

Analysis of the character 濡 *rú*

Consists of three parts.

- Left: reduced form of 水 *shui* = water
- Top right: rain falling from the sky
- Bottom right: a plant
- Character as a whole: gives the idea of dampness, but also softness (like cooked meat). The classic description of this pulse is a thread in the water.

Characteristics

- Forceless
- Thin
- Felt at the superficial level
- Delicate – can easily be occluded

Causes

This pulse may indicate the presence of external Dampness. It may also result from Qi, Blood or Yin deficiency, which makes Yang unrooted and ascending to the surface.

Wave contour

slippery   choppy   overflowing   stirring

 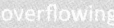

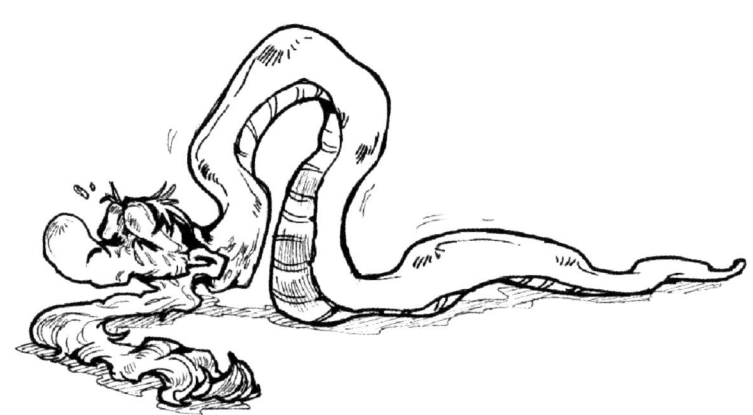

Normal pulse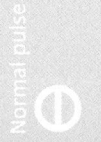

Width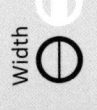

Length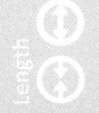

Depth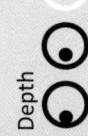

Speed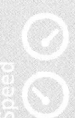

Rhythm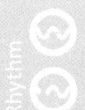

Strength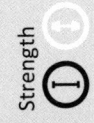

Vessel wall tension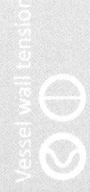

弱脈 *ruòmài* – Weak pulse

Analysis of the character 弱 *ruò*

Shows two wings of a yang bird with feathers, resembling the shape of bows. It is a picture of a yang bird's plumage, which is delicate, weak, fragile.

Characteristics

- Forceless
- Thin
- Delicate – can easily be occluded
- Felt at the deep level

Causes

This pulse characterizes a weak constitution. It may also indicate Qi (especially Yang Qi) and Blood deficiency.

Wave contour

| slippery | choppy | overflowing | stirring |

Vessel wall tension

The wall of the vessel reflects the state of Qi, especially the Yang aspect of Qi.

Increased wall tension

Increased wall tension is caused by Qi stagnation.

Pulses with increased wall tension:

→ *xianmai*

→ *jinmai*

→ *gemai*

→ *koumai*

→ *shimai*

→ *laomai*

⊘ Decreased wall tension

Qi and Blood deficiency cause decreased wall tension.

Pulses with decreased wall tension:

→ *sanmai*

→ *weimai*

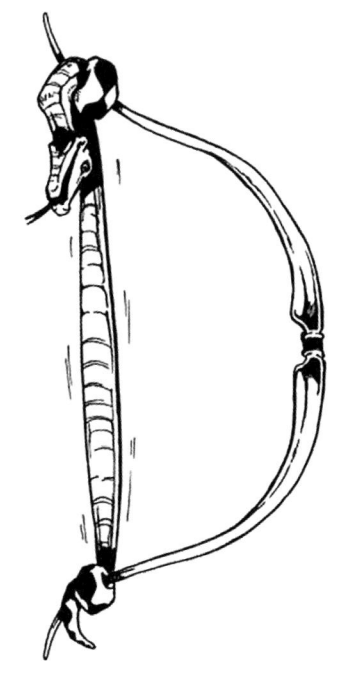

Normal pulse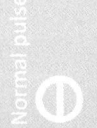

Width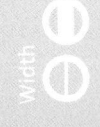

Length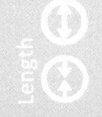

Depth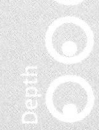

Speed

Rhythm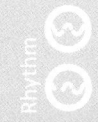

Strength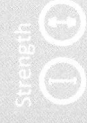

Vessel wall tension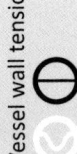

弦脉 *xiánmài* – Wiry (stringlike) pulse

Analysis of the character 弦 *xián*

Consists of two parts.

- Left: arrow

- Right: thread

- Character as a whole: a tensed bowstring or a tensed string of a musical instrument

Characteristics

The wiry pulse is defined by increased wall tension. Because of that the vessel cannot easily be occluded by increased finger pressure.

Causes

The increased wall tension reflects Qi stagnation, which may be caused by:

- disturbances of the Wood element (Liver, Gallbladder)

- pain

- presence of Dampness and/or Phlegm

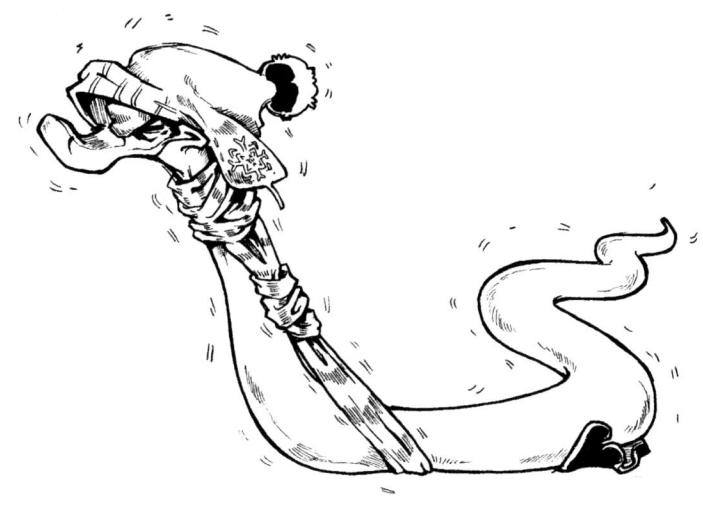

Normal pulse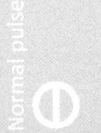

Width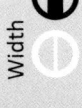

Length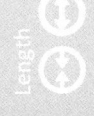

Depth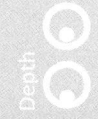

Speed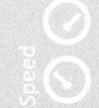

Rhythm

Strength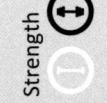

Vessel wall tension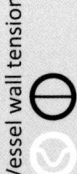

緊脈 *jǐnmài* – Tight pulse

Analysis of the character 緊 *jǐn*

Consists of three parts.

- Top left: minister
- Top right: hand; together giving the idea of an official who firmly rules his staff, and in a wider sense symbolizing firmness and solidness
- Below: silk
- Character as a whole: tight binding

Characteristics

- Increased wall tension
- Increased strength
- Trembling which gives an impression of increased width

Causes

The tight pulse is typical for the presence of Cold. It may also appear when there is pain and food stagnation.

Wave contour

slippery   choppy   overflowing   stirring

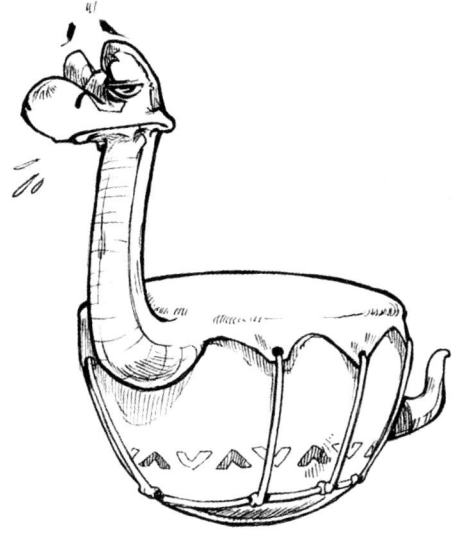

Normal pulse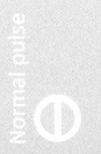

Width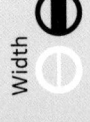

Length

Depth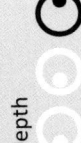

Speed

Rhythm

Strength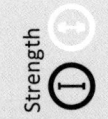

Vessel wall tension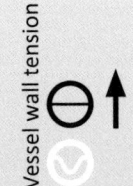

革脈 *gémài* – Drumskin pulse

Analysis of the character 革 *gé*

The Chinese character depicts streched out, raw sheep skin, meaning a skin which is stretched for example on a drum.

Characteristics

- Significantly increased vessel wall tension
- Increased width
- Decreased strength
- Being felt strongest at the superficial level
- Susceptibility to occlusion under strong pressure of fingers – impression of emptiness inside

Causes

In situation of fluid loss, when the vessel cannot be filled, a sudden attack of Cold can cause significant tension of the vessel wall, and the ascending of the pulse towards the surface.

This pulse image may also result from a sudden loss of large quantities of fluids (including Blood). Uncontrolled Yang makes the pulse ascending to the surface, and causes tension of the wall; deficient substances are not able to fill the vessel.

The difference between *gemai* and *koumai* refers to the intensity of the wall tension.

Wave contour

slippery 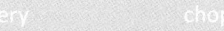 choppy overflowing 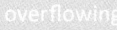 stirring

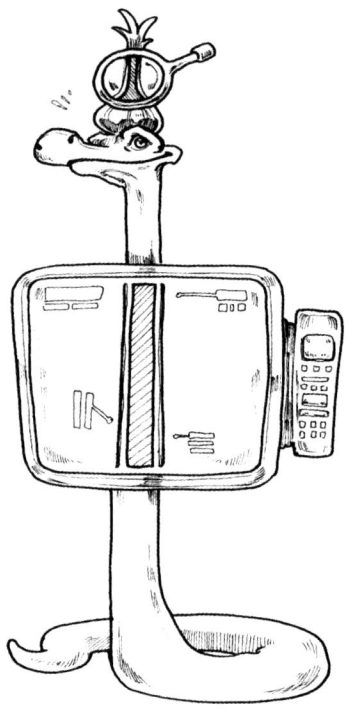

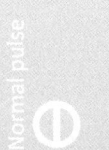 Normal pulse

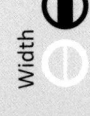 Width

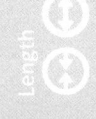 Length

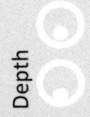 Depth

 Speed

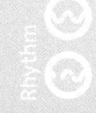 Rhythm

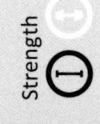 Strength

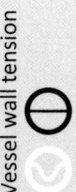 Vessel wall tension

芤脈 *kōumài* – Hollow pulse, scallion pulse

Analysis of the character 芤 *kōu*

Consists of three parts.

- Above: characters for grass

- Bottom left: child

- Bottom right: swallow; both together show the picture of a swallow feeding its brood. Because swallows build their nests in holes in Chinese mud houses, these two characters give an idea of something which is empty, hollow.

- Character as a whole: a plant which is hollow, like a scallion, spring onion

Characteristics

- Slightly increased wall tension

- Increased width

- Decreased strength

- Being felt strongly at the superficial level

- Being easily occluded, but even then the wall is felt

Causes

Hollow pulse reflects Yang without Yin. Such a situation may happen in case of loss of Blood, when the pulse is hollow and empty, or in case of Yin deficiency, when the pulse is hollow and accelerated.

The difference between *gemai* and *koumai* refers to the intensity of the wall tension.

Wave contour

slippery   choppy   overflowing   stirring

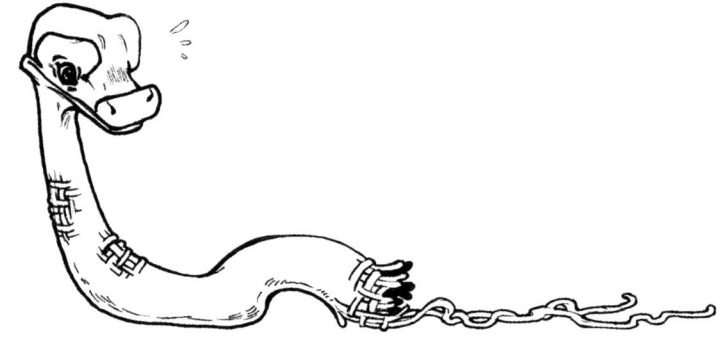

Normal pulse

Width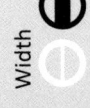

Length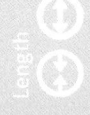

Depth

Speed

Rhythm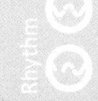

Strength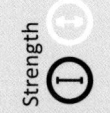

Vessel wall tension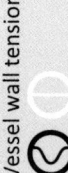

散脉 *sǎnmài* – Scattered pulse

Analysis of the character 散 *sǎn*

Consists of three parts.

- Top left and bottom: meat fibers

- Right: a hand holding a rod

- Character as a whole: chopping up a piece of meat that dissolves into fibers; symbolizing 'scattering', 'dissipating', 'dispersing'

Characteristics

- Decreased tension of the vessel wall, there are no clearly detectable boundaries

- Decreased strength

- Increased width

- Being strongly felt at the superficial level

- Being very easily occluded

Causes

The scattered pulse is a result of serious Qi and Blood deficiency, when Yang deficiency causes decreased wall tension and strength, and Yin deficiency leads to a lack of filling the vessel, which enables easy occlusion. This pulse may also be a result of Yuan Qi deficiency.

Wave contour

slippery ●●●

choppy ‿‿‿‿‿‿

overflowing

stirring

Speed

Speed is mainly a reflection of the state of Yang Qi as a Blood moving force.

⊘ Increased speed

Increased speed is caused by Yang hyperactivity:

- presence of Yang pathogens
- internal Heat
- Yin deficiency

Fast pulses:

→ *shuomai*

→ *jimai*

→ *cumai*

→ *dongmai*

Decreased speed

If Yang activity is insufficient, the speed will decrease. The reasons for this are:

- presence of Cold
- Yang deficiency

Slow pulses:

→ *huanmai*

→ *chimai*

→ *jiemai*

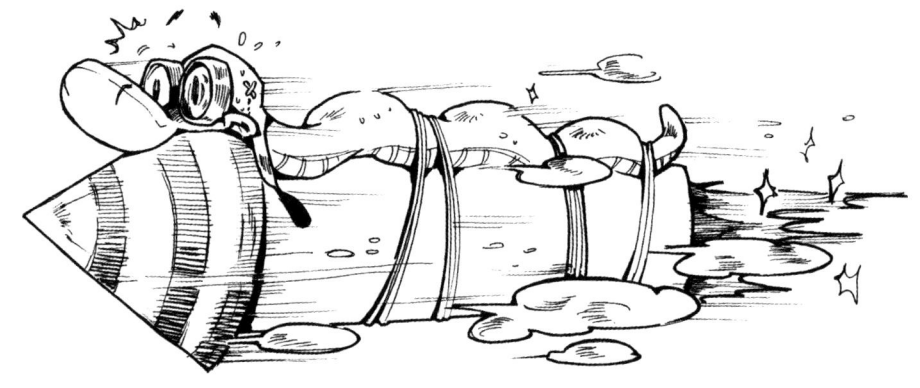

Normal pulse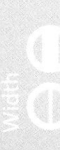

Width

Length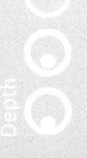

Depth

Speed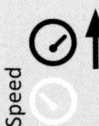

Rhythm

Strength

Vessel wall tension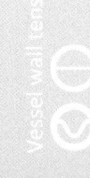

疾脉 *jímài* – Racing pulse

Analysis of the character 疾 *jí*

Consists of two parts.

- Outside: a man lying in bed, meaning 'illness'
- Inside: 矢 *shi* = arrow
- Character as a whole: urgent situation, such as a serious disease

Characteristics

The racing pulse is very fast – defined by more than seven heartbeats per one in-breath.

Causes

A racing pulse may result from Yin exhaustion (in which case it is racing and weak) or presence of excessive Heat (in which case it is racing and strong).

The situation of the patient is serious in both cases.

Wave contour

slippery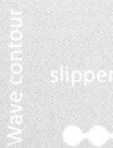

choppy

overflowing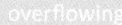

stirring

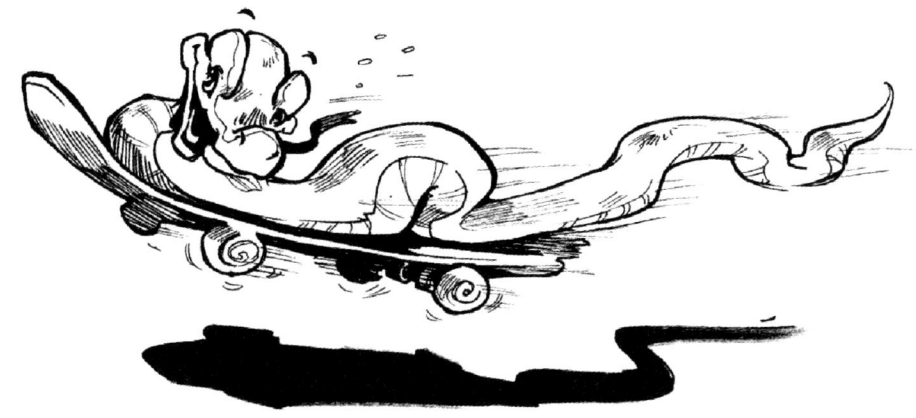

 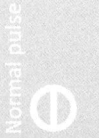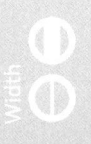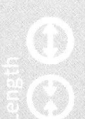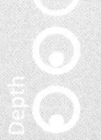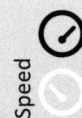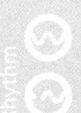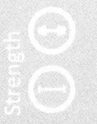

數脈 *shuòmài* – **Fast pulse, rapid pulse**

In modern Chinese *shuo* means 'frequently', 'often' or 'rapidly'.

Analysis of the character 數 *shuò*

Consists of two parts.

- Left: an imprisoned woman

- Right: a hand holding a rod

- Character as a whole: idea of governing and authority

Characteristics

A fast pulse is faster than normal, and defined by more than five heart-beats per one in-breath.

Causes

Speed is a function of Yang Qi, so a fast pulse is the result of Yang excess (in that case the pulse is fast and strong) or a fast pulse can be the result of Yin deficiency (in that case the pulse is fast and weak).

When there is sudden loss of Blood the pulse may become fast and hollow.

Wave contour

slippery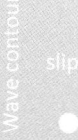

choppy

overflowing

stirring

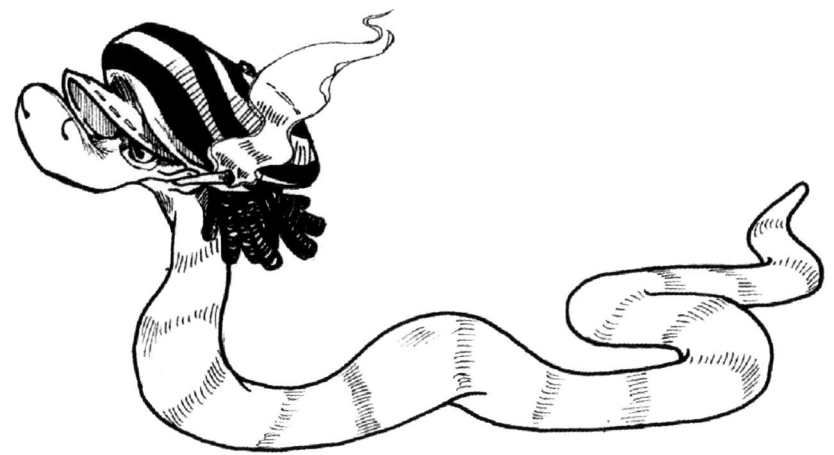

Normal pulse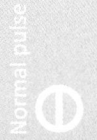
Width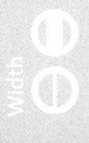
Length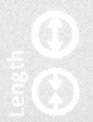
Depth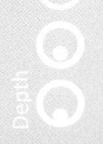
Speed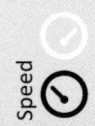
Rhythm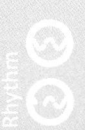
Strength
Vessel wall tension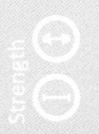

緩脈 *huǎnmài* – Relaxed, moderate pulse

Analysis of the character 緩 *huǎn*

Consists of two parts.

- Left: radical for silk thread

- Right: balance, pause

- Character as a whole: smooth balanced thread (or pulse)

Characteristics/causes

huanmai is considered as being physiological by many authors. Its Chinese name may also indicate this. Nevertheless it tends to be defined as slightly slower and more slippery than normal. In the latter case it may be a result of Qi deficiency and presence of Dampness.

Wave contour

slippery   choppy   overflowing   stirring

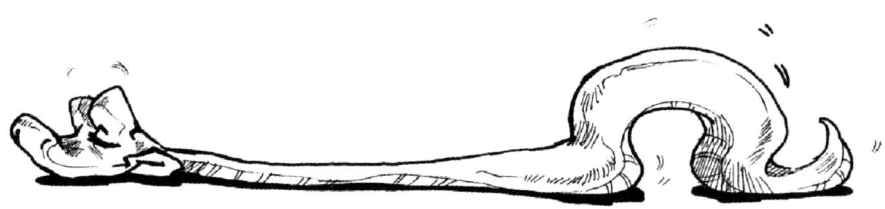

Normal pulse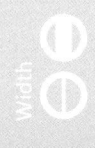

Width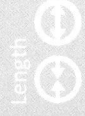

Length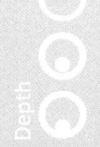

Depth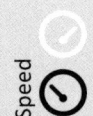

Speed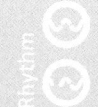

Rhythm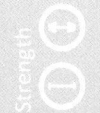

Strength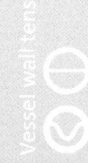

Vessel wall tension

遲脈 *chímài* – Slow pulse

Analysis of the character 遲 *chí*

Consists of two parts.

- Left: radical for 'walking'

- Right: Tibetan yak

- Character as a whole: the slow walk of this big animal

Characteristics

The slow pulse is slower than normal, being defined by less than four heart-beats per one breath.

Causes

Speed is a function of Yang Qi, so the slowing down of the pulse indicates Yang deficiency (in that case the pulse is slow and weak) or the presence of Cold (in that case the pulse is tight and slow). It may also be observed in athletes, in which case it is not a disharmony.

slippery   choppy   overflowing   stirring

Wave contour

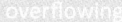

Rhythm

The Rhythm of the pulse reflects mainly the state of Heart Qi, and is proof of the Shen being present in the pulse. That is why processes disturbing Shen (pain, fright) influence the rhythm. Moving is a Yang function, so changes in rhythm may be caused by excesses of Heat and Cold, and also tumors and masses.

Regular breaks in the rhythm

Rhythm disturbances, or pauses in rythym can be regular, which means that from a series of heartbeats some are missing.

Regularly interrupted pulse:
→ *daimai*

Irregular breaks in the rhythm

An irregularly interrupted pulse may be either faster than normal (in the case of deficiencies of Yin aspects, or excess of Yang) or slower than normal (in the case of deficiencies of Yang aspects or excess of Yin nature). The speed is a factor which allows a differentiation of irregularly interrupted pulses.

Irregularly interrupted pulses:

→ *cumai*

→ *jiemai*

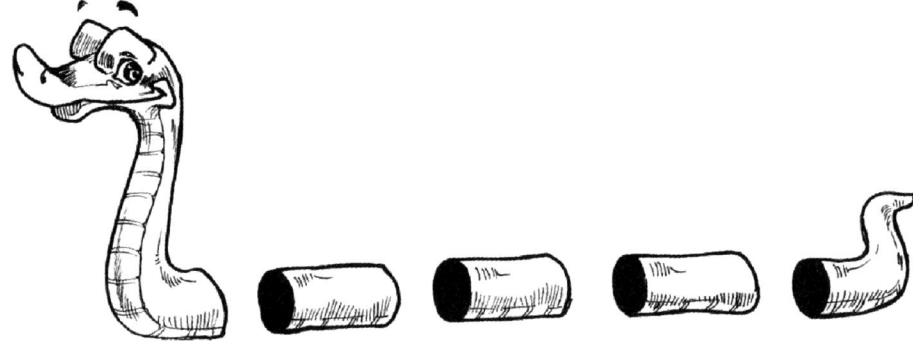

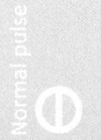
Normal pulse

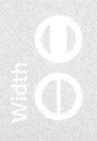
Width

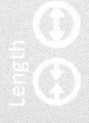
Length

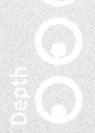
Depth

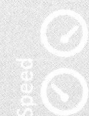
Speed

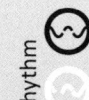
Rhythm

Strength

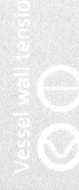
Vessel wall tension

代脈 *dàimài* – Intermittent pulse

Analysis of the character 代 *dài*

Consists of two parts.

- Left: a man

- Right: a pin that was used to count things

- Character as a whole: series, sequence or succession; for the pulse this indicates a problem with the rhythmical sequence of heartbeats, gaps in a pulse sequence

Characteristics

The intermittent pulse is defined by regular gaps in rhythm.

Causes

Rhythm is related to Heart Qi. This pulse may be caused by exhaustion of Heart Qi and may be associate with congenital defects, dystrophies or damage such as fevers and infarction. Yuan Qi deficiency, and Jing Qi deficiency will result in the presence of an intermittent pulse.

This pulse may be also present due to severe pain and emotional shock disturbing Shen, and when there is Qi and Blood stagnation.

Wave contour

slippery

choppy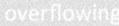

overflowing

stirring

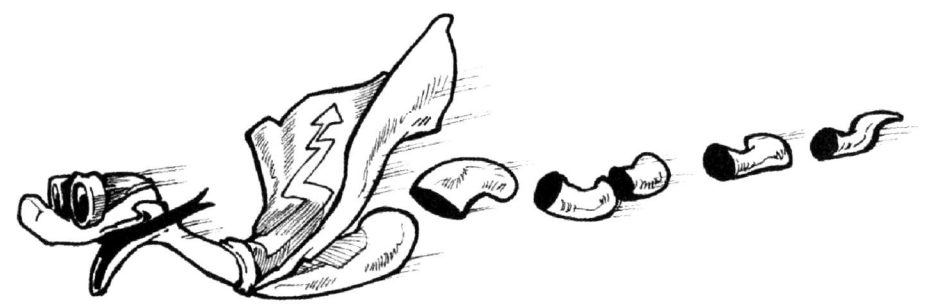

Normal pulse

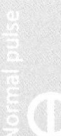

Width

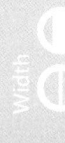

Length

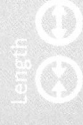

Depth

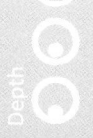

Speed

Rhythm

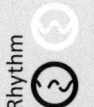

Strength

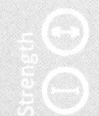

Vessel wall tension

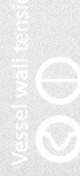

促脈 *cùmài* – **Skipping pulse**

Analysis of the character 促 *cù*

Consists of two parts.

- Left: a man
- Right: a foot
- Character as a whole: a man hurrying, haste

Characteristics

- Irregular gaps in rhythm
- Increased speed

Causes

This pulse may result from exhaustion of Heart Qi and Blood or exhaustion of fluids, or Fluids exhaustion. It may also be a consequence of Qi stagnation and subsequently created Heat accelerating the pulse.

Wave contour

slippery   choppy   overflowing   stirring

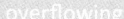

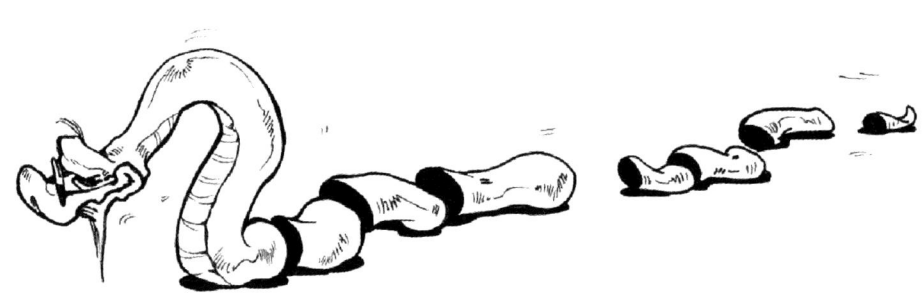

Normal pulse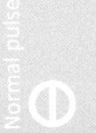

Width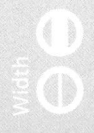

Length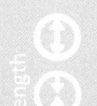

Depth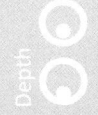

Speed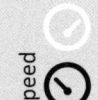

Rhythm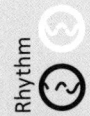

Strength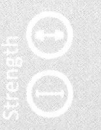

Vessel wall tension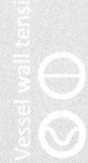

結脈 *jiémài* – **Knotted pulse**

Analysis of the character 結 *jié*

Consists of three parts.

- Left: radical for silk thread
- Top right and bottom: happiness, luck, related to marriage
- Character as a whole: happy knot

Characteristics

- Irregularly interrupted
- Slower than normal

Causes

This pulse may be created when there is Yang Qi and Yuan Qi deficiency. Also excesses of Yin aspects, such as Cold, or accumulations and masses may slow down the pulse and block the vessel leading to an irregular pulse.

slippery

choppy

overflowing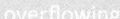

stirring

Wave Contour

In contrast to simple parameters, which were discussed previously, wave contour is a pulse quality describing a complex set of feelings concerning blood flow through a vessel.

If blood flow is felt as smooth, as a roundish shape moving through a vessel, the pulse is called slippery.

Turbulent blood flow results in a rough pulse.

If the pulse is like a spinning bean (short, strong, fast), the pulse is called stirring.

A shape similar to a wave which hits a cliff with strength and goes weak, defines a surging pulse.

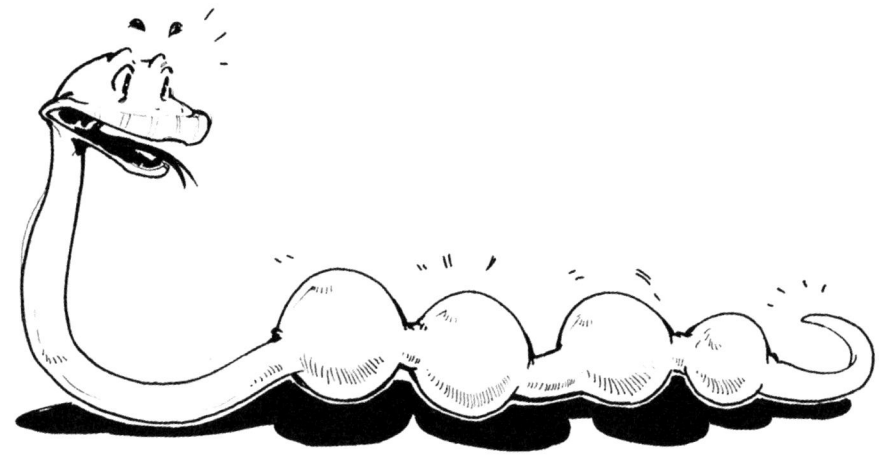

Normal pulse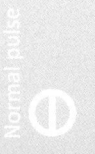

Width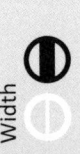

Length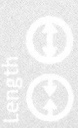

Depth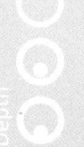

Speed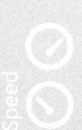

Rhythm

Strength

Vessel wall tension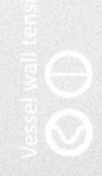

滑脈 *huámài* – Slippery pulse

Analysis of the character 滑 *huá*

Consists of two parts.

- Left: reduced form of 水 *shui* = water

- Right: 骨 *gu* = bones

- Character as a whole: something polished, smooth, which refers to the impression of this pulse

Characteristics

In the classics this pulse is compared to pearls rolling in a bowl. The feeling of this pulse resembles a roundish, rather soft shape thrusting its way through the vessel, extending it from the inside. For this reason the pulse may be considered as wide.

Causes

When there are no signs of disease, a slippery pulse may indicate a state of health. A specific type of this pulse may be felt in pregnant women at the *chi* position.

A slippery pulse may result from:

- presence of Dampness, including food stagnation (the shape reflects stagnation)

- presence of Heat (Fire energy extends a vessel from inside)

Wave contour

| slippery | choppy | overflowing | stirring |

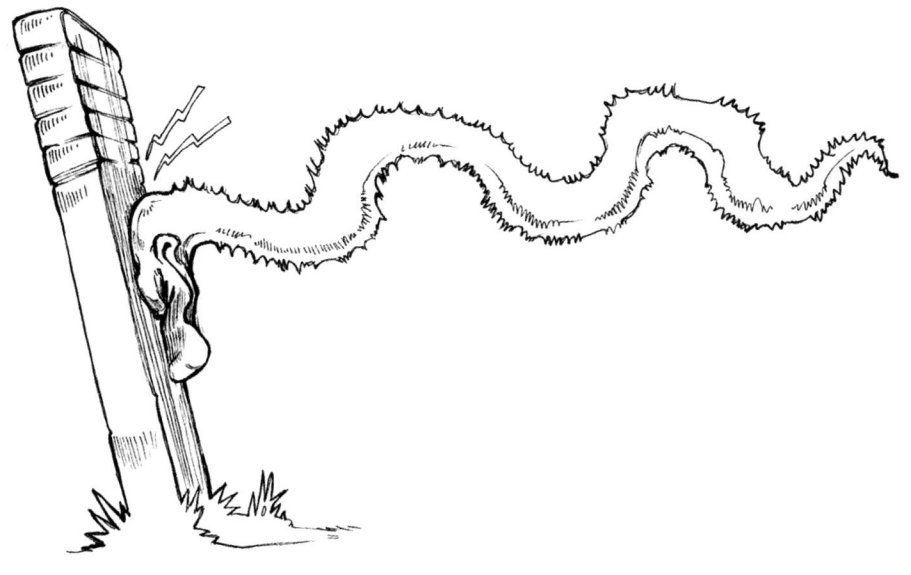

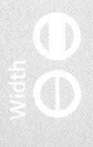 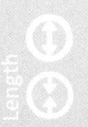 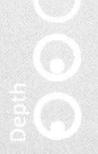 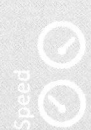 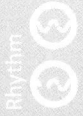 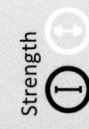

Normal pulse

Width

Length

Depth

Speed

Rhythm

Strength

Vessel wall tension

澀脈 *sèmài* – Choppy, rough pulse

Analysis of the character 澀 *sè*

Consists of five parts.

- Left: reduced form of 水 *shui* = water
- Above (double): sharp edged weapon, like a knife
- Below (double): marching or stopping
- Above and below together: a rough or irregular surface, which obliges many steps in various directions
- Character as a whole: water being scattered while dropping onto the sharp edge of the knife

Characteristics

The choppy pulse is similar to the feeling of an arteriovenous fistula (for example in dialysis patients), the pulse is 'buzzing' like a running transformer.

Causes

The choppy pulse indicates turbulent Blood flow. It may be a result of:

- Deficiencies of Yin aspects (deficiencies of Blood, Jinye or Jing)
- Qi and Blood stagnation
- Food stagnation or presence of Phlegm

Wave contour

slippery   choppy   overflowing   stirring

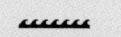

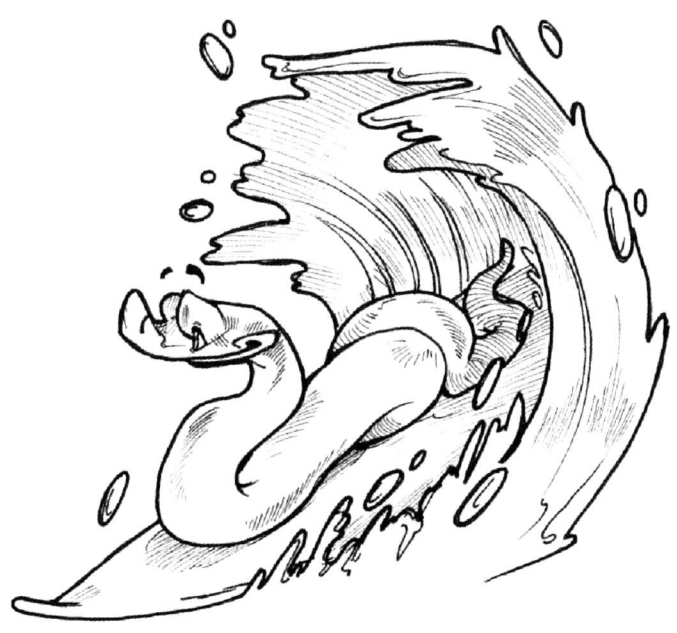

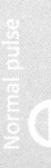
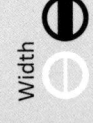
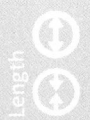
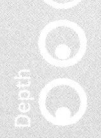
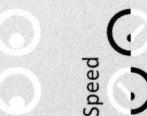
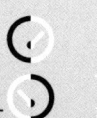

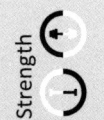
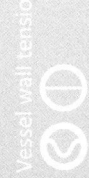

洪脈

hóngmài – Surging, overflowing pulse

Analysis of the character 洪 *hóng*

Consists of two parts.

- Left: reduced form of 水 *shui* = water

- Right: an act carried out together

- Character as a whole: flood or large amount of water

Characteristics

- Big

- Wave-like: it comes strong and goes away weak

Causes

Yangming is abundant of Blood and Qi. A pathogen in Yangming leads to big, strongly expressed symptoms. One of the symptoms is the surging pulse.

Wave contour

slippery

choppy

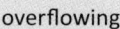

overflowing

stirring

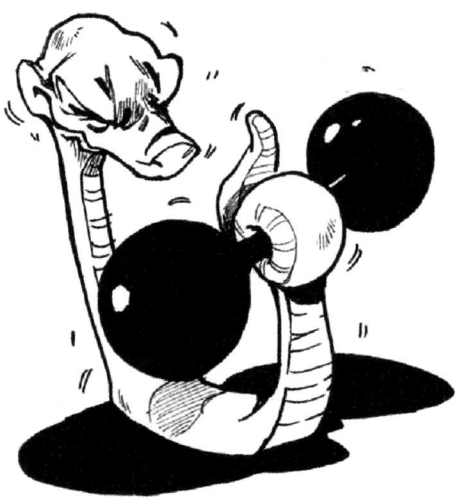

Normal pulse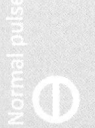

Width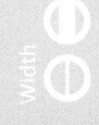

Length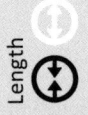

Depth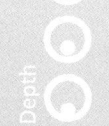

Speed

Rhythm

Strength

Vessel wall tension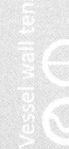

動脈 *dòngmài* – Stirring pulse

Analysis of the character 動 *dòng*

Consists of two parts.

- Left: a man lifting something heavy from the ground; 'heavy'. Mostly used for defining repetition of action with great effort.

- Right: tensed sinew

- Character as a whole: a movement (possibly repeated) done with great effort

Characteristics

The stirring pulse tends to be compared to a spinning bean, and is defined as:

- short

- strong

- fast

Causes

The stirring pulse may result from:

- presence of Heat

- trauma

- pain

- fright

Wave contour

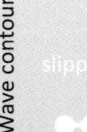

slippery

choppy

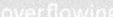

overflowing

stirring

Overview of all pulses

	Icon	Pulse illustration	Chinese	Name	Excess	Deficiency
Width			細脈	ximai	Dampness	↓ Qi and Xue, ↓ Jinye
Depth			浮脈	fumai	Presence of pathogen (pulse floating and forceful)	↓ Yin (pulse floating and forceless)
			沉脈	chenmai	Pathogen inside (pulse deep and forceful), Qi and Xue stagnation	↓ Yang Qi (pulse deep and forceless), ↓ Xue (pulse deep and forceless)
			伏脈	fumai	Yang Qi stagnation caused by food stagnation or deep penetrating pathogen (pulse hidden and forceful)	↓ Yang Qi, serious (pulse hidden and forceless)
Length			長脈	chang-mai	Internal Heat, rising Liver Yang	
			短脈	duanmai	Qi stagnation (pulse short and forceful)	↓ Qi (pulse short and forceless)
Strength			實脈	shimai	External pathogen fighting with strong Wei Qi, stagnated Heat leading to Fire, toxic Heat	
			牢脈	laomai	Pathogen deep, cold penetrating the inside (stomach, intestines, uterus), Qi and Xue stagnation	
			虛脈	xumai		↓ Qi
			微脈	weimai		↓ Qi and Xue (chronic, serious), shock, Yang collapse
			濡脈	rumai	External dampness	↓ Qi and Xue, or Yin
			弱脈	ruomai		↓ Qi (Yang Qi) and Xue, weak constitution
Vessel wall tension			弦脈	xianmai	Liver and Gall Bladder disorders, dampness or phlegm, pain	
			緊脈	jinmai	Cold, pain, food stagnation	

Icon	Pulse illustration	Chinese	Name	Excess	Deficiency	
⊖↑ ◑ ○ ⊖		革脈	gemai	Sudden attack of cold (when ↓ Jinye)	Sudden serious loss of fluids, chronic disease leading to serious ↓ Yin and Jing	Vessel wall tension
⊖ ◑ ○ ⊖		芤脈	koumai		Loss of Xue (pulse hollow and forceless), ↓ Yin (pulse hollow and fast)	Vessel wall tension
⊘ ◑ ○ ⊖		散脈	sanmai		↓ Qi and Xue (serious form), ↓ Yuan Qi	Vessel wall tension
⊘↑		疾脈	jimai	Heat and Yang hyperactivity (pulse racing + forceful)	↓ Yin (pulse racing and forceless)	Speed
⊘		數脈	shuomai	Heat (pulse fast and forceful)	↓ Yin (pulse fast and thin), ↓ Xue (pulse fast and hollow)	Speed
⊘		緩脈	huanmai	Dampness	↓ Spleen Qi	Speed
⊘		遲脈	chimai	Cold (pulse slow and forceful)	↓ Yang (pulse slow and forceless)	Speed
⊗		代脈	daimai	Qi and Xue stagnation, strong pain, emotional shock	Exhaustion of Heart Qi, ↓ Yuan Qi/Jing Qi	Rhythm
⊗ ⊘		促脈	cumai	Heat and stagnation	Exhaustion of Jinye, exhaustion of Heart Qi and Xue	Rhythm
⊗ ⊘		結脈	jiemai	Free flow of Qi and Xue to heart blocked by cold, masses and tumors	↓ Yang Qi, ↓ Yuan Qi	Rhythm
slippery ◑		滑脈	huamai	Health, pregnancy, food stagnation, dampness, heat		Wave contour
choppy, rough ⊖		澀脈	semai	Qi and Xue stagnation, food stagnation, phlegm	↓ Yin – Jinye, Xue, Jing	Wave contour
overflowing, sirging ⊘ and ⊘ ⊖ and ⊕		洪脈	hongmai	Pathogen on Qi level/Yangming		Wave contour
stirring ⊕ ⊘ ⊕		動脈	dongmai	Heat, trauma, pain, fright		Wave contour

Sources to the explanations of the Chinese characters

Internet pages active at the time of the publication of this book:
http://chinese-characters.org
http://www.rtega.be/chmn/
http://www.chineseetymology.org

Bibliography:
Li Leyi, Tracing the roots of Chinese characters:
500 cases, Beijing 1993

Index

KIENER PRESS

Joy of Learning

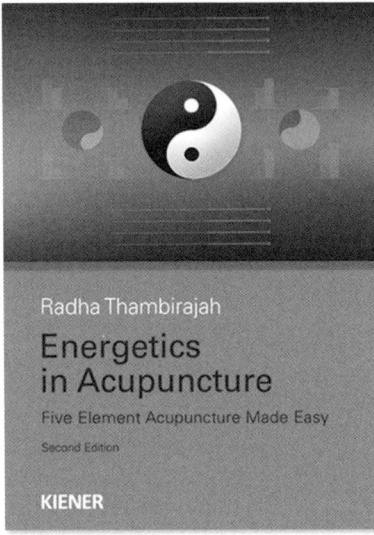

Radha Thambirajah

Energetics in Acupuncture

Five Element Acupuncture
Made Easy

2nd edition 2018
464 pages
100 illustrations
Softcover, 17 x 24 cm
ISBN 978-3-943324-53-2

Energetics in acupuncture provides a
simple diagnostic method to find out
which aspects of Qi are out of balance
and which acupuncture treatment is
required. Once the correct diagnosis
has been made, the relevant points can
be treated with appropriate techniques.
The book follows a logical approach to
diagnosis and provides relevant questions
and conclusions.

- Treatments are described for over
  80 different diseases.
- Innovative visual "towers" clearly
  show what an energy imbalance looks
  like
- Case studies illustrate unbalanced
  states.

KIENER PRESS

Joy of Learning

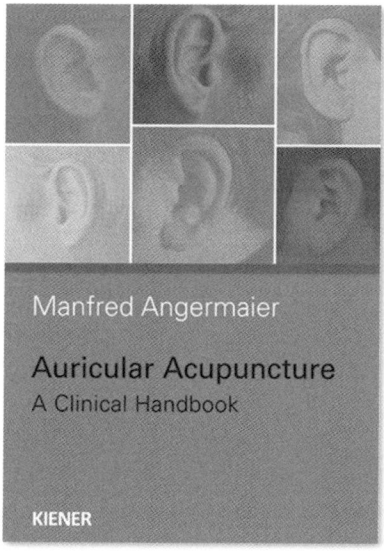

Manfred Angermaier

Auricular Acupuncture
A Clinical Handbook

1st edition 2014
432 pages
200 illustrations
Hardcover, 14,8 x 21 cm
ISBN 978-3-943324-29-7

Translated from German into
English by Johanna Schuster

The author explains in this guide how a wide range of disorders and diseases can be treated with various point combinations.

This book is a translation of "Leitfaden Ohrakupunktur" (Elsevier).

- Quick orientation through illustrations of the ear points and information on localization and indication, presented on double pages
- Point recommendations for pain therapy and many other diseases
- Case studies which demonstrate the therapeutic strategy in words and pictures.

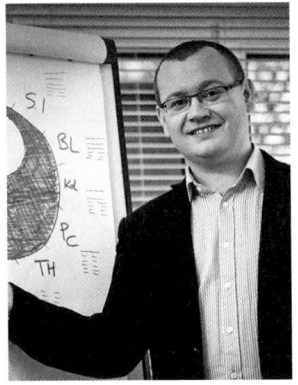

Bartosz Chmielnicki is a doctor and has been working with acupuncture since 2004. Together with Dr. Michal Richter, he founded a center for natural medicine – Compleo and Silesian Academy of Acupuncture – Compleo. He is the co-author of the curriculum for basic acupuncture training for doctors in Poland.

He was president of the Silesian Chapter, an association of the Silesian Technical University, board member of the Polish Acupuncture Association from 2007–2009, and president of the Society for Classical Acupuncture from 2010–2014.

He works as an acupuncturist at Compleo in Katowice and cooperates with the pain clinic of the clinic in Tychy. He likes to share his knowledge and experience with colleagues and organizes basic and advanced training courses at the Silesian Acupuncture Academy, Compleo.

He also holds seminars on acupuncture and participates in postgraduate studies in pain management for doctors organized by the Colledium Medicum of the Jagiellonian Universities in Kraków. He is a recognized teacher in other countries and gives courses and lectures at congresses and conferences in Poland, the Czech Republic, Israel and Germany – including the TCM congress in Rothenburg o.d.T.

He is the author of articles, book chapters, posters and a book on pulse diagnosis. He works with Dr. Yair Maimon and Rani Ayal on a project on the clinical use of acupuncture points.